MOTHER'S FIRST TIME PREGNANCY GUIDE: What to anticipate throughout pregnancy and delivery.

Nathan C. Jolly

TABLE OF CONTENT

INTRODUCTION

You're about to become a mother—congrats! Being a parent is exciting and terrifying all at once. Future parents may experience a range of emotions, including joy, pride, dread, concern, and insecurity. These emotions are all normal. This is a critical period for both you and your partner. As you embark on this novel and thrilling journey known as parenthood, you will need each other's support and inspiration.

When you have a baby, especially your first, a lot of things change. The majority of first-time parents have no idea what to anticipate from the significant occasion or how the new child would affect their life.

You'll need to learn how to balance your family, work, and education commitments. In addition to new joys and worries, your new baby will also come with new pressures. It's common to experience some degree of overwhelm.

You shouldn't expect to understand everything right away. In how you feel, you are not alone. This transitional period will end.

Future mothers Are in the best possible health!

- Eat nutritious foods. Eat several servings of whole grains, fruit, vegetables, and foods high in calcium and protein, such as milk, yogurt, and cheese, each day. Limit your intake of salty, sugary, and fatty foods.

- Eat foods high in folate (the natural form of folic acid), such as green leafy vegetables, kidney beans, orange juice, peanuts, broccoli, asparagus, and peas, and take a folic acid supplement. Bread, pasta, rice, and cereal are enhanced foods with folic acid. Folate aids in the production and maintenance of healthy cells in the body, which is crucial for pregnant women.

- Keep moving. Include physical activity in your everyday routine. You can reduce stress and have a healthy pregnancy by exercising. To build the ideal workout program for you, consult your doctor.

- Remain psychologically sound. Although having a baby is a great event, there will occasionally be stress involved. Parenting seems to go better for people who feel good about themselves. Be sure to give yourself space to unwind and cope with stress. Your baby is at risk if you smoke, drink, or use drugs.

Chapter 1

HOW YOU'RE FEELING

As it gets ready to develop a new life, your body is about to go through some significant changes.

You can begin to feel symptoms like nausea or weariness, or you might discover that you have more energy than usual! Pay attention to your body's signals and modify your exercises as necessary. Every pregnancy is unique, just like every woman.

Early pregnancy indicators and symptoms
For women who experience menstruation on a regular monthly basis, a missed period is the first indication of pregnancy.

Implantation hemorrhage might happen occasionally. This bleed resembles a light period or spotting a lot. Even though this is totally natural, if you feel any bleeding while you are pregnant, you should consult your doctor.

Some of the symptoms listed below, such as exhaustion, nausea, or more frequent urination, may also appear early in your pregnancy.

ordinary signs

Your entire body is affected by the hormone changes that occur during the first few weeks of pregnancy. While every pregnancy is unique, some signs you could encounter in the first trimester include:

Breast sensitivity

Extreme mood swings Vomiting or nauseousness (morning sickness)

often urinating

Loss or increase of weight

extreme tiredness

Headaches

Heartburn

Leg twitches

pelvic and lower back pain

a desire for particular foods

newfound aversion to some meals

Constipation

Taking care of oneself

To put it mildly, early pregnancy symptoms can be painful. After consulting your doctor first, consider these suggestions for some relief. Always base your decisions on your preferences and the options that are accessible to you.

Try ginger, chamomile, vitamin B6, and/or acupuncture for nausea or vomiting.
Try calcium or magnesium if you get leg cramps.
If the dietary changes advised by your healthcare physician are not alleviating your constipation, you may get comfort from wheat bran or other fiber supplements.
For the duration of your pregnancy, eating well and exercising frequently are essential. As long as it's comfortable for you, keep up your everyday physical exercise. You will adjust to your changing physique more readily if you are more active during pregnancy. Make careful to feed nourishing nourishment to the developing bodies of

both you and your infant. Make sure you are consuming a range of healthy foods, such as vegetables, meat, beans, nuts, pasteurized dairy, and fruit, to ensure that you are getting enough energy, protein, vitamins, and minerals.

Chapter 2

HOW YOUR BABY IS GROWING

The most essential time for your baby's development is right now. Your baby's physique and internal organs are developing during the first trimester. Early body and organ development includes:

spine and brain

Inside ear

heart tissue

Genitals

Fingernails

Liver\sEyelids

Pancreas

Kidneys

the hands, feet, and limbs' cartilage

the muscles in the nose, eyes, and mouth

fingers and toes with webs

Lungs

For a variety of reasons, fetal growth can vary greatly, but during the first trimester, your baby will grow from approximately 0.64 cm (.25 in) at the end of the first month (smaller than a grain of rice) to approximately 10 cm (4 in) by the end of week 12 and will weigh approximately 28 g. (1 oz) [Data from Cleveland Clinic] Please consult your country's ministry of health for information.

When should I schedule a consultation with my doctor?

During your first 12 weeks of pregnancy, you should make at least one appointment with your doctor; ideally, do so as soon as possible. Please contact your nation's health ministry or a medical facility for recommendations.

Chapter 3

THINGS TO LOOK OUT FOR

Even if every pregnant woman has a unique pregnancy experience, you should consult your doctor if you encounter:

cervical spotting During the early stages of pregnancy, spotting known as implantation bleeding can be common; but, in certain situations, spotting or bleeding may be caused by a more dangerous condition, such as an ectopic pregnancy, a molar pregnancy, or a cervical infection. If the spotting is heavy and is followed by other symptoms like shoulder discomfort, severe dizziness, or abdominal or pelvic pain, call your doctor.

severe or persistent vomiting Both nausea and vomiting might be perfectly normal first-trimester symptoms. Although it's more generally referred to as "morning sickness," it doesn't always manifest in the morning. The unusual disease is known as hyperemesis gravidarum, which necessitates medical care, and maybe the cause of your extreme morning sickness if it is accompanied by other symptoms like dizziness or bloody vomit. If you suffer vomiting after the first trimester, speak with your doctor to rule out anything serious and get the nausea under control.

burning while urinating or the need to go. A urinary tract infection may be present if you experience an increased need to urinate but just a few drops come out or if you experience burning when urinating (UTI). Fever, chills, and blood-tinged urine are some other signs of a UTI. To prevent problems, your physician will be able to identify your symptoms and treat the bacterial infection. Remember that during the first trimester and later in pregnancy, as your baby grows and puts pressure on your bladder, frequent urination on its own is a typical pregnancy symptom.

faintness or dizziness Early on in the second trimester, feeling dizzy can be a common symptom. Later on in your pregnancy, you could experience vertigo as a result of issues with your blood circulation or low blood sugar. Consult a medical professional, though, if the dizziness is persistent, you feel faint or do faint, or if it is accompanied by other symptoms like headaches, nausea, or pain in your belly, or impaired vision, so that a reason may be found and treated.

Mid-to-Late Pregnancy Symptoms You Should Pay Attention to:

lower abdominal discomfort It's normal to be concerned about abdominal pain while pregnant. Remember that discomfort brought on by, say, round ligament soreness may be completely natural. When you cough or sneeze, this will feel like a dull discomfort or a sharp pain on either side of your belly. However, stomach pain that is perhaps accompanied by a fever or chills could be a clue that something is wrong. It would be better to speak with your healthcare practitioner in this situation.

A beating heart Your heart should beat more quickly while pregnant. In actuality, compared to when you are not pregnant, your heart pumps up to 30 to 50% more blood. This is done to ensure that your baby gets the right amount of nutrients and oxygen through the placenta. However, get in touch with your healthcare physician right away if you believe your heart rate is continuing to be elevated and/or you are experiencing shortness of breath.

a terrible headache Numerous variables, including hormone changes, stress, and weariness, might contribute to headaches during pregnancy. But if your headache is unbearably bad, it can be an indication of high blood pressure or preeclampsia, a hazardous illness that can develop after 20 weeks of pregnancy or even after giving birth. To save both your and your unborn child's health, medical intervention is necessary.

Alterations to eyesight. Vision changes, including momentary blindness, impaired vision, or sensitivity to light, may be related to conditions like prenatal hypertension or preeclampsia.

edema or puffiness, and unusual weight gain. Preeclampsia is associated with sudden, significant weight increase that is not the result of overeating. You may have noticed that this weight gain is also accompanied by edema, or swelling, of the hands and face. Keep in mind that minor swelling in your hands or feet may be normal, but it should still be watched.

severe ache under the ribs and above the stomach. Preeclampsia, a related condition with high blood pressure, and stomach pain during pregnancy may both be present (particularly if they coexist with additional symptoms like nausea, headaches, or impaired vision). During prenatal checkups, your healthcare practitioner will check your blood pressure, but if you detect any preeclampsia symptoms, call your provider straight away.

vaginal dripping. More vaginal discharge than you did before becoming pregnant will be present. Changes in your cervix and vagina might result in this discharge, which is typically sticky, clear, or white. However, if the color is not clear or white, if it smells unpleasant, and if it is accompanied by pain, soreness, or itching, you may have a vaginal infection. For a diagnosis and treatment, speak with your healthcare professional.

lower back ache. In the latter stages of your pregnancy, lower back pain is typical. After all, your body is coming closer to giving birth, and your pelvic ligaments are loosening to facilitate the baby's entrance. The sciatic nerve is compressed by your expanding uterus, which can also result in lower back pain from sciatica. Your lower back, hip, and back of the leg may hurt in this situation. Contact your doctor if you also experience numb feet, weakness in one or both legs, or if your calf is painful.

less frequently feeling your baby move Sometime between 18 and 25 weeks of pregnancy, women frequently start to feel the baby moving, kicking, or turning. Your doctor might ask you to keep count of how long it takes you to feel 10 kicks, rolls, or flutters if you're well into the third trimester. If an hour goes by without any movement, eat a little snack, lie back down, and try again. It might only take a few minutes. These movements can be recorded in a notebook. Call your doctor to make sure everything is going properly if you notice a lack of movement or if your baby isn't moving as much as usual over the days.

uterine bleeding It's crucial to inform your healthcare professional as soon as possible if you experience bleeding throughout the third trimester because it can develop into a major problem. Instances of placenta previa, in which the placenta covers the cervix, or placental abruption, in which the placenta starts to split from the uterine wall, can also cause bleeding.

All-over itching The condition known as cholestasis of pregnancy, a liver disorder that can happen in late pregnancy, may cause severe itching that isn't accompanied by a rash. If you experience extreme itching, speak with your healthcare professional straight away. Keep in mind that itching skin during pregnancy is very normal. This is because as your baby grows, your skin will expand and may also become dry, which may make itchy regions like your belly, breasts, and thighs.

Preterm contractions are contractions that occur before 37 weeks of pregnancy. If your contractions persist (i.e., don't stop when you move or change positions) and become painful or regular, it may be an indication you are in preterm labor. However, these sensations can also be completely typical Braxton Hick's practice contractions. It's crucial to speak with your healthcare practitioner right away in this situation.

Fluid gushing or trickling from your vagina (before the end of 37 weeks of pregnancy). Before your pregnancy is fully developed, your "water breaking," also known as an early rupture of the membranes, may appear as a trickle, a constant leak, or a torrent of fluid from your vagina. If you see this, contact your healthcare professional straight away. Your water breaking once you have reached full term indicates that labor has begun.

Vaginal discharge or spotting (between weeks 37 and 40 of pregnancy). Light spotting or a pink or barely bloody discharge could occur. As the cervix has started to dilate and the mucus plug that had been sealing it off has started to loosen, this can be an early symptom of labor. However, if the bleeding is severe, get in touch with your doctor right once.

Bottom Line

Keep in mind that while some of these symptoms may be typical during pregnancy, they also could indicate a more serious condition. For the most suitable advice, speak with your healthcare professional.

Consult your provider if you have any questions or if something doesn't seem right. In this manner, you won't have to worry, and if a problem does arise, it can be resolved right away.

www.ingramcontent.com/pod-product-compliance
Lightning Source LLC
LaVergne TN
LVHW020543160826
845677LV00015B/4181

9798361450480